DRAW ME A GIRONDA

RAW EGG NATIONALIST

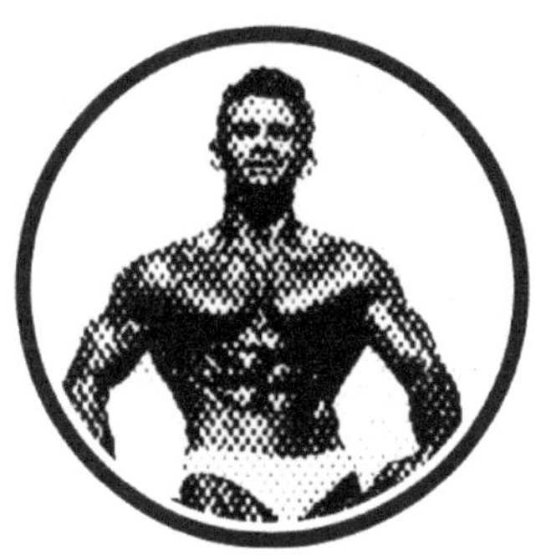

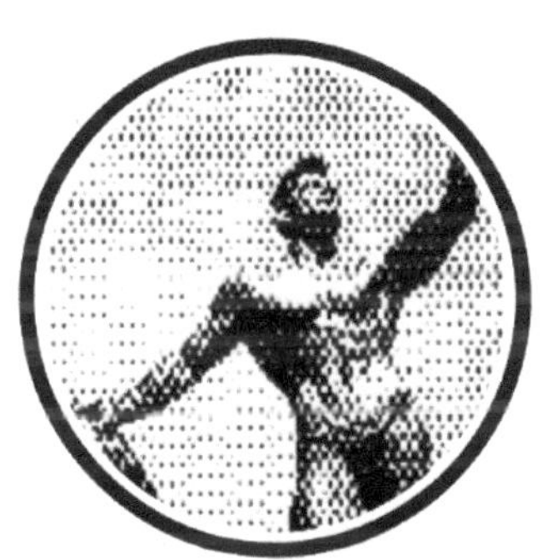

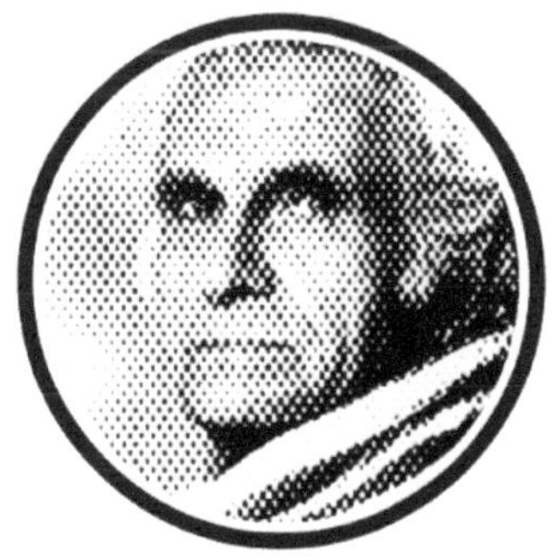

-Hey. Can I ask you to do something for me?

-Umm. Depends what it is?

-Can you draw me a Gironda?

-A Gironda!?

-You know, like, Vince Gironda. The Iron Guru. Owner of Vince's Gym. Inventor of the drag curl and the 8x8. Called Arnold a fat fuck.

- Oh my god, I love him! Gimme a minute.

I wait. Ten minutes later, she sends me the picture. It's Vince Gironda all right. In just a few moments, I know everything I need to know about her. This, my friends, might be the start of something beautiful…

The next time you match with a girl on Tinder or Bumble, ask her to draw you a Gironda. Go on. Do it. It will tell you things about her that might otherwise take some time to come to light. It might tell you things she'll do her best to hide; better to learn them now rather than months or years down the line, amirite?

Is she creative?

Impatient?

Generous?

The Gironda she draws will tell you that.

Does she have daddy issues?

A prior DUI?

A nasty drug habit?

Yes, her Gironda will tell you that as well. You might even say that the Iron Guru is a Love Guru too…

This book will tell you everything you need to know about drawings of Vince Gironda and how to interpret them. As well as providing general guidelines for interpreting them, there will be a selection of examples of Girondas I've encountered in the wild, with a detailed commentary on each of them. At the end, you'll even have the chance to draw your own Gironda and see what it says about you.

First, though, I suppose I should tell you a little about the man himself.

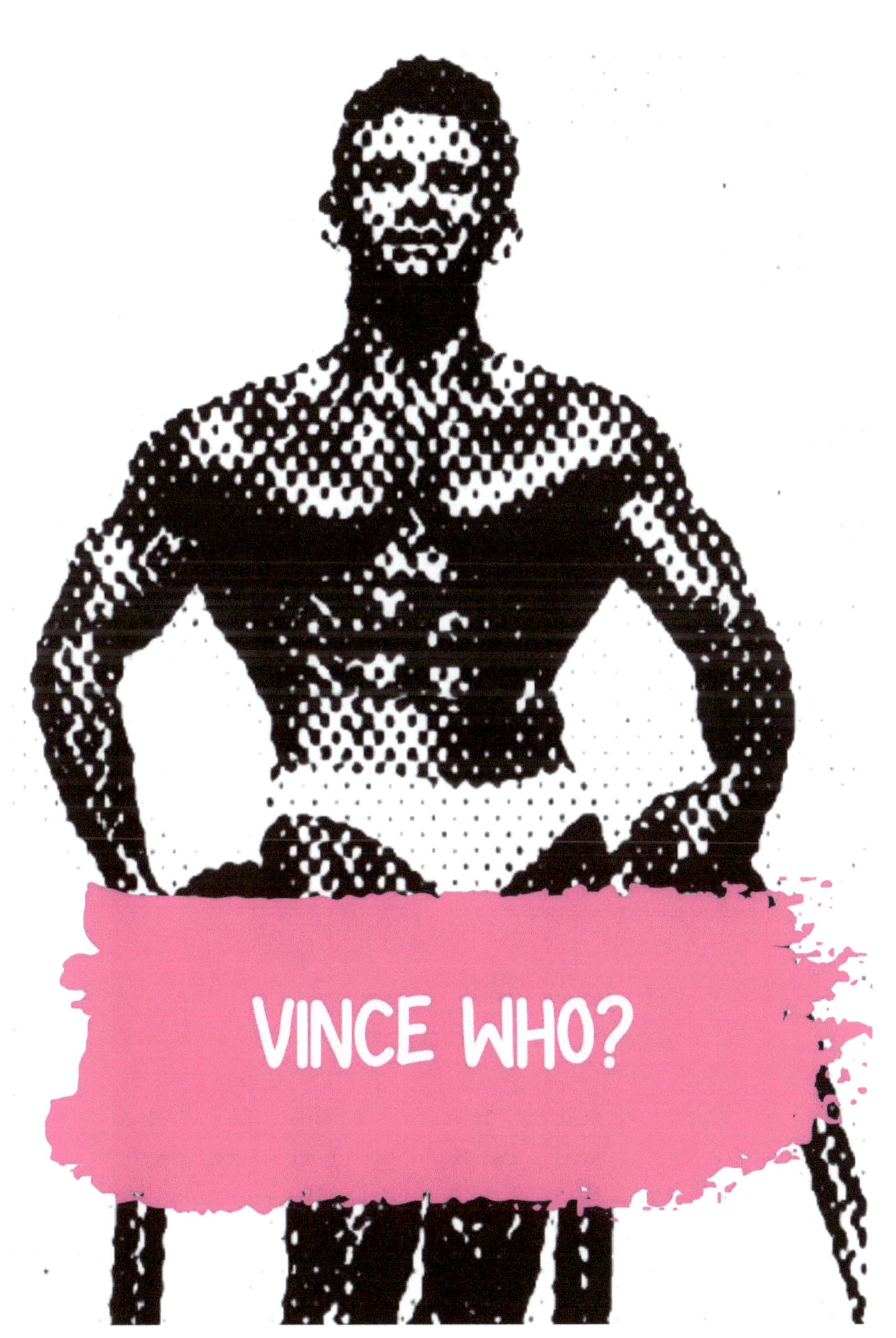
VINCE WHO?

On Twitter once I referred to Vince Gironda as the 'Nikola Tesla' of bodybuilding. If you know anything about Nikola Tesla, the great inventor and futurist, you'll understand what I'm getting at. Tesla was a brilliant maverick whose contributions to the furtherance of knowledge and indeed the human spirit have been unfairly overlooked, even suppressed; a man well before his time (they say the Trump family knows his secrets...). So it is for Vince Gironda too. If a lot of what I am going to say to you seems familiar – about ketogenic dieting and fasting, for instance – that's because Vince was talking about and advocating such things decades before your favourite Instagram or YouTube fitness 'expert'. And if, as T.S. Eliot put it, 'the end of all our exploring will be to arrive where we started and know the place for the first time', a proper account of the history of bodybuilding and of fitness culture more generally will have to recognise the contributions of men like Vince Gironda, and the many paths that could have been taken but weren't. Things could have been very different.

Vince embodied a truly experimental approach to bodybuilding, one that was informed not only by his own personal experience of developing muscle for aesthetic purposes, but also by the latest scientific and historical papers of his time. He was also famous for his frank speech, and his refusal to praise the unpraiseworthy – an admirable trait which in any age never fails to go unpunished. Indeed, one of his most famous workouts is known as the 'Honest Workout'. But for every Arnold who was spurred to train harder and achieve more by being called a 'fat fuck' by Vince, there must be dozens who weren't; many were expelled from his gym simply for asking why there weren't any squat racks or why there wasn't any music playing. Bodybuilding changed massively in his lifetime too, from the classically proportioned physiques of men like Steve Reeves and Vince himself, to the mass monsters of the early 1990s, like Dorian Yates.

So, for many years, Vince fell by the wayside, his ideas about diet and his routines were forgotten, or claimed by others as their own. In recent years, however, he has enjoyed something of a revival, especially due to the fast-growing populist movement known as Raw Egg Nationalism, which has harnessed Vince's famous 36-eggs-a-day diet to an anti-globalist political stance. Here is Vince's story, in my words – and with a few of his own thrown in for good measure.

THE STORY IN OUTLINE

'There's no doubt about it – I am hated and I am loved. Why? Because I am dogmatic. I have this unforgivable feeling inside me that when it comes to bodybuilding I know what I'm talking about. If it ruffles feathers, so be it. I can neither compromise to save feelings nor stretch the truth to flatter and please. I am my own man – egocentric, controversial, and proud.'

After spending the first seven years of his life living in the Bronx, the young Vince Gironda moved with his family to Los Angeles in the early 1920s. His father worked as a stuntman on a number of Hollywood films, including *Ben Hur* (1925), the most ambitious and the most expensive silent film ever made. The first movie stuntmen were true daredevils, including large numbers of rodeo riders and actual cowboys, who were put to good use in the burgeoning western movie scene. The demands and the dangers of the job, long before the days of CGI, were legendary, and so it was expected that these men should be not just brave but also extremely fit. Little is known about Vince's father's background, apart from that he was not much of a weightlifter, unlike many of his fellow stuntmen. Vince himself was more interested in dance during his early years, until his father 'persuaded' him to return to the fold of more traditional masculine pursuits. (I can't help but picture the scene as Billy Elliot meets Tony Soprano, with exactly the result you'd expect. 'My son a fuckin' dahncer!?')

Unlike Chuck Sipes and Chet Yorton, two of the Golden Age bodybuilders I wrote about in my previous book, Vince displayed serious promise as a young athlete, setting local records in various running events as well as pole vaulting. Eventually, he decided to follow in his father's footsteps and become a stuntman. Realising he might need to pack on a little muscle to do so, Vince joined the local YMCA gym. At the age of 23, he had his mind blown by a photograph of John Grimek, 'the Monarch of Muscledom', a bodybuilder who was also an early inspiration to Reg Park. Grimek won the Mr America in that year (1940) and the next, and went on to win the Mr Universe in 1948, in London, before winning the 1949 Mr USA and then retiring undefeated. Like many bodybuilders of that time, Grimek was also a serious strength competitor, having represented the US at the 1936 Olympics, in Berlin, where he placed 9th. Grimek's dominance of the nascent bodybuilding scene was so great that after his second win a new rule was made preventing previous winners of the Mr America from competing again. His other nickname, 'the Glow', was coined in reference to how brightly he stood out on stage in contrast to his competitors.

When he first started training, Vince weighed 148lb, some 40lb less than he would eventually weigh, with 12" arms, a 39" chest and 20" thighs. After eight months of serious bodybuilding training at the YMCA, he moved to Harvey and Dale Easton's gym in West Hollywood, which has been described as one of the first 'dungeon gyms' in Los Angeles and is still open today. The gym was an early favourite for bodybuilders and Hollywood celebrities alike. The Easton brothers themselves were responsible for the invention of the preacher curl machine and other exercise equipment. Vince was put on an intensive weight training course and made significant gains. He went on to work as an instructor at the gym for a year, during which time he was able to continue his experimentation with muscle-building methods.

Soon it became clear that Vince was on to something with his own training ideas, and with the encouragement of his clients he decided to open his own gym. Vince's Gym, at 11262 Ventura Blvd., opened in 1948; it would remain open for 40-something years, through the most transformational period in bodybuilding history. At the time of its opening, Vince's Gym was only one of two dedicated bodybuilding gyms on the west coast, the other being Jack La Lanne's gym in San Francisco; on the east coast, there was also Sig Klein's gym, where Reg Park would train when he visited the US in preparation for his first Mr Universe win, in 1951.

Vince and his eponymous gym were an immediate success. Easily the most notable of the early successes was with 'the Golden Boy' Larry Scott, the man who would win the very first Mr Olympia contest, in 1965, and along with Reg Park and Bill Pearl become one of the sport's first crossover stars.[1] After winning the Mr Idaho competition in 1959, Scott moved to California to train. Vince took him under his wing and helped him further build and refine his physique, including turning a weak point, his biceps, into his strongest through the use of preacher curls. With Vince's help, Scott became the first bodybuilder to boast 20" arms. His work ethic was legendary – he worked out for two hours a day, six days a week – and one of the main reasons Vince was prepared

---

[1] Scott's other mentor was Irving Johnson, more commonly known as Rheo Blair, one of the early pioneers of protein supplementation. I talk about Rheo Blair, and his protein shakes below, as well as in *Raw Egg Nationalism in Theory and Practice*.

to invest as much time in him as he needed to be a champion. And a champion he soon was. In 1960 he won the Mr California, followed by Mr Pacific Coast the next year; in both contests he also won the 'most muscular' prize. Mr America followed in 1962, and Mr Universe in 1964. The inaugural Mr Olympia contest, which Scott won in 1965, was established by the Weider brothers to sort the best from the best of all the many competing federations of the time: only winners of the Mr America or Mr Universe competition could participate. Scott won the Olympia the next year too, and then retired, much to the shock of the bodybuilding community, to focus on other projects.

After Larry Scott, Vince would train a succession of the sport's best, including Don Howarth, Frank Zane, Lou Ferrigno and Arnold Schwarzenegger; the influence he had on these legends would be more than enough, in itself, to guarantee his place in the annals of the sport. Arnold, in particular, came to Vince at a difficult time, after the second of two losses that would prove transformational for his career; in his book, *Muscle, Smoke and Mirrors*, Randy Roach describes this period as 'Arnold's Cuban Missile Crisis'. The first of the two losses, which I discuss in my previous book, *Three Lives of Golden Age Bodybuilders*, was to Chet Yorton in the 1966 Mr Universe in London. Arnold first met Vince two years later, when he was about to compete in the 1968 Mr Universe. He entered Vince's Gym in fine spirits, confident of his upcoming victory, and telling everybody who would hear; Vince, however, didn't share his optimism, and casually dismissed the young Austrian as a 'fat fuck'. Two weeks later, after losing the Universe title to Frank Zane, Arnold returned and was forced to admit that Vince had been right. Up to that point, Arnold had not paid much attention to his diet, but now under the tutelage of Vince – for whom bodybuilding was, in his own words, '85 percent nutrition' – he was able to elevate his conditioning. Arnold eventually won Vince over with his work ethic, which Vince described as a 'slow, plodding Germanic type of drive'.

Arnold had to look elsewhere, however, to increase his knowledge of the latest performance-enhancing drugs. From the beginning, Vince was always opposed to drug use, not only on ethical grounds but also because he believed steroid use only produced puffy, swollen bodies – the opposite of the kind of well-proportioned bodies he championed. An entire chapter of his most famous training manual, *The Wild Physique* is titled 'Steering Away from Steroids'. 'I detest the use of chemicals by any athlete in any sport', he writes.

'Everything about drugs rubs me the wrong way. Unlike many pro bodybuilders who see benefits that outweigh the disadvantages, I see only the atrocious side effects... and absolutely *no benefits*.'

In his final interview before his death in 1997, Vince asked 'whatever happened to physical culture?' His answer was stark: 'In a bodybuilding world gone mad, it no longer exists.' He pointed to the use of human growth hormone in particular, which was probably first used in the early 1980s, if Dan Duchaine's 'underground steroid handbook', dating to 1982, is a reliable guide. Other practices he decried included intramuscular injections, 'producing an instant increase in size without loss of definition' and the use of cosmetic surgery.

As well as operating Vince's Gym, Vince of course trained and competed in bodybuilding shows himself, through the 1950s and into the 1960s. A year after opening the gym, he placed fourth in the 1949 Mr California. Two years later, he finished second in Mr America. Despite the obvious quality of his physique, he would never win a major title, his best result being second place in Class II of the 1962 NABBA Mr Universe. In many instances, Vince suffered for being *too ripped*, at a time when a softer, rounder musculature was preferred.

Vince's favourite diet to get in optimal shape for competition was called the 'Maximum Definition' diet, which was basically a ketogenic diet. The diet involved eating steak and eggs three times a day, and nothing more (except a selection of supplements, including Vince's favourites: liver tablets and kelp tablets); carbohydrate consumption was limited to once every four days. I will talk about this diet later in more detail, when I discuss Vince's routines and diets.

But it wasn't just hardcore bodybuilders who sought out Vince Gironda and his famous training methods. Like at the Eastons' gym, Hollywood celebrities were regularly to be seen at Vince's Gym, especially after his success with Larry Scott. It became clear to Hollywood executives looking to get their leading men in screen-worthy shape that Vince was the man to turn to. A full list of celebrities Vince had trained up to 1984 is included as the final chapter of his book, *The Wild Physique*, with his thoughts on each of them, some quite surprising. He noted Cher's sense of humour; David Carradine's introversion; Clint Eastwood's 'quiet charisma' – a 'fun-loving rowdy'; Marty Feldman's love of talking about 'soccer and world politics'; Kurt Russell's initial grudging acceptance of having to work out; Shawn Penn's studiousness; Carl Weather's almost unlimited physical potential – 'What a natural!... An Olympic athlete or an Olympia bodybuilder – both are within his grasp'.

Vince capitalised on the success he had as both a bodybuilding and a celebrity trainer by publishing extensively. As well as writing his own pamphlets – with such titles as 'A Muscle Has Four Sides', 'Balanced Arms', 'Blueprint for the Bodybuilders', 'How I Train the Stars' and 'Secrets of Definition' – he wrote a regular column for *Iron Man* magazine which earned him his moniker of 'the Iron Guru'. He also had a mail-order business which included nutritional supplements under the brand NSP Nutrition. The publication of his 1984 book, *The Wild Physique*, written with *MuscleMag International* publisher Robert Kennedy, was followed by a promotional tour in which Vince gave seminars throughout North America to packed audiences.

By the early 1990s, however, Vince's fortunes were on the wane. This was due both to his son Guy's worsening health, which took up more and more of Vince's time, and to the changing nature of the fitness industry. Guy had been a regular helper at Vince's Gym, but appears to have developed a serious drug habit; little information about him, or the exact nature of what ailed him, is to be found. The general movement of bodybuilding and the fitness industry more generally had been away from rather than towards Vince's own ideas, and a gym that had been fit for purpose and among the best equipped in the 1950s and 1960s was no longer so 30 years later. Vince's Gym suffered by comparison with newer, larger and better equipped gyms that opened in the area; not that Vince thought so himself, however ('I would never install a piece of apparatus that I didn't think would help a person build a great physique'). In his final published interview, he lamented various changes that had made it harder to run an honest fitness business, including rampant steroid abuse, corruption in the bodybuilding federations and an increasing desire for 'certified' trainers. He told an amusing story about how one of his female clients had actually dropped Don Howarth – a former Mr America with 40 years of bodybuilding experience – because she learned that he was not 'certified' as a trainer. Disregarding Howarth's 'uncertified' advice about the way she was training her back, she had soon injured herself and had to give up training. Vince's Gym closed in 1995. Vince died two years later.

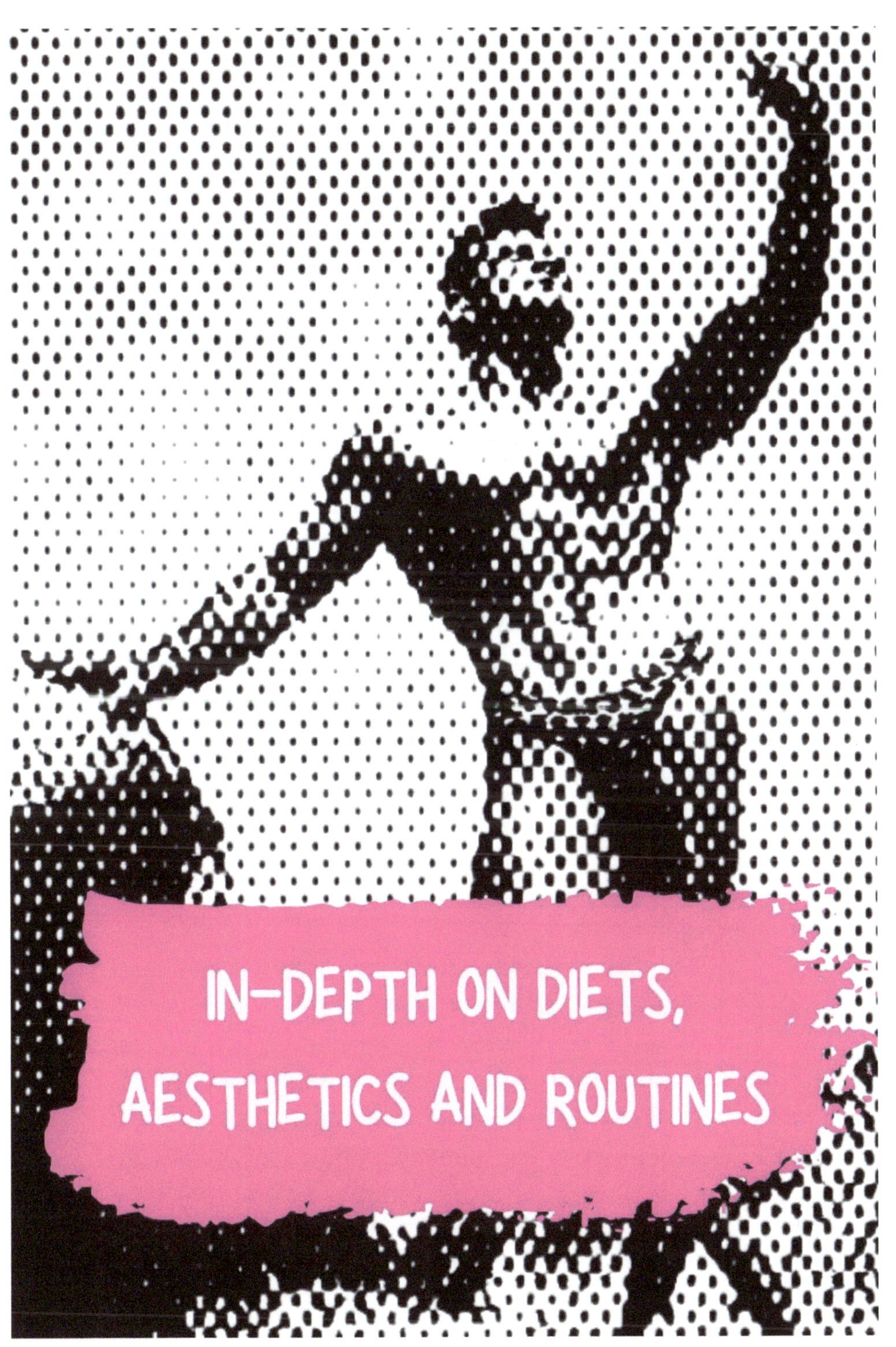
IN-DEPTH ON DIETS,
AESTHETICS AND ROUTINES

An account of Vince Gironda's life would of course be incomplete without a discussion of the aesthetic ideas, diets, exercises and routines that made him who he was; Vince was an innovator and a freethinker on every front. It would be impossible in a slim volume such as this to do full justice to the range of ideas that Vince had over the course of some five decades in bodybuilding and fitness, so I'll stick to what I consider the most important and interesting ideas.

Vince's emphasis was always on aesthetics as opposed to the mere cultivation of mass which has led, in our day, to such freakish physiques as those of the 'mass monsters', starting with Dorian Yates. 'Since when was a work of art judged merely by its hugeness?' Vince asked. He was in no doubt that the human body was, or should be, a work of art, and therefore should be judged by the standards of art.

> 'The human body is God's greatest creation. I believe that its development should be *maximized*, but always with respect for the individual's skeletal and genetic potential. I do not believe in overcrowding the frame to the extent that the individual is all bunched up, unable to walk

correctly. Muscle has to be placed on the frame with care.'

It shouldn't be a surprise, then, that when this aesthetic standard of mass for art's sake was finally abandoned for mass for its own sake, Vince himself and his teachings were largely forgotten. If Vince had addressed himself to a bodybuilder like Mike Mentzer, he would almost certainly, as Ron Kosloff has suggested, have told Mike the following: ease off the back squats, because of your over-developed arse and hips (pipe down back there, Rippetoe!); reduce your heavy ab work and narrow your bulky waist; and stop working your traps so much, because you are losing perceived width in your already relatively narrow shoulders. For Vince, creating an aesthetically pleasing physique was as much about 'illusion' as anything else. Even if you don't have naturally wide shoulders, as Mike Mentzer or indeed Larry Scott didn't, you can still make it appear that you do; but to do so you must exercise the intelligent, discerning and ultimately dispassionate eye of the artist.

On the whole, instead of focusing on the traditional mass building compound movements, Vince favoured isolation movements, which was in line with his principle that mass must be added as carefully as possible to the body, in the right proportions and the right places. As a result, there were certain exercises, among them the back squat, which Vince discouraged; indeed, in his own gym, they were fully *verboten*. Owing to his belief that back squats lead to overdevelopment of the glutes and widening of the hips, Vince's Gym famously had no squat racks; in *The Wild Physique*, he even stated that asking for a squat rack to be installed in his gym had led to members being expelled (one of at least 12 sacred laws not to be violated, other examples of which are given below). Instead of using squats as the primary leg developer, Vince recommended leg extensions and curls, hack squats and an exercise known as the 'sissy squat', which is anything but for sissies. Although the sissy squat is credited to Vince, it was actually probably invented by Monty Wolford, another bodybuilder of the Golden Age. The squat takes place in three phases. Stand with your feet about a foot apart, with your heels on a 2" block and a light barbell held at the shoulders in the clean position. Drop down with a straight back, keeping your shoulders over your heels, and then back up once you have reached the lowest position. Next go into a full squat, on your heels, then thrust the hips forward until the body and thighs form a straight line with the shoulders, before sitting back on the heels. Finally, raise yourself to standing. The three phases together count as one rep.

Other popular exercises Vince hated included the traditional bench press, which he claimed involved too much front deltoid and not enough chest. Instead, he recommended doing weighted dips, but with a grip distance of 32″ to ensure that most of the work is done by the chest, or doing a variation of the bench press dubbed the 'guillotine press', which involves taking a much wider grip on the bar and lowering it to the neck, rather than the chest. According to Vince, Larry Scott was able to build his Olympia-winning chest by alternating dips and guillotine presses – and nothing else. Vince also disliked high-rep ab work and especially sit-ups, which he believed were totally ineffective, because the work is done mainly by the psoas major, a back muscle, and not the rectus abdominis; he claimed sit-ups lead only to lordosis (curving of the lumbar spine). Instead, Vince preferred a type of crunch he called, aptly for us internet anons, the 'frog crunch'. Lie on your back and draw your heels back and under your hips, like a frog. Holding a plate behind your head, curl your head and upper body down, bringing your chin to your chest, so that only your lower back remains on the floor. Hold the contraction for two seconds, then return to the starting position.

Vince was an absolute believer in the power of intention, intensity and the importance of the much vaunted, but generally elusive, mind-muscle connection. This was one reason why, on the whole, he shunned complicated machines in favour of free weights, incline benches and a few simple pieces of machinery, like the hack press machine. Despite regularly being offered 'large chrome machines' by every equipment company, he declined all such offers: 'with machines there is no curiosity aroused. Movement can only be done one way. The experience is not creative, hence boredom sets in for the mind and muscles.' For similar reasons, music of all varieties was banned from Vince's Gym. (Vince's Gym was perhaps the closest we have come to realising Plato's Republic, at least in that regard.) 'Music is only useful to hype and control the tempo and cadence of aerobic-type exercises which are done at a lively dance pace. In addition, everyone's taste in music is different.' People who asked for music to be played 'appear to have no concept of the mental state that must be achieved to succeed in bodybuilding.' A swift and permanent exit from the gym usually followed.

As far as fuller routines go, Vince created a wide variety with different rep schemes. In his book, *The Wild Physique*, he expressed his preference for doing eight sets of eight (8x8): this is the 'Honest Workout' I mentioned earlier. Vince believed the routine was not for a beginner.

'I call it the "honest workout" because of the pure muscle fibre that can be attained with this combination. Keep to 8x8 and your muscle fibre will plump out, giving you a solid mass of muscle density as a result.'

For the 8x8, a good starting weight would be one you can lift 10-12 times. Vince generally cautioned that the amount of reps and sets you do should ultimately depend on your 'training frequency and recuperation time'. Intensity 'should always be over 85% to trigger growth'; the number of sets you need to achieve maximum stimulation of the muscle 'is directly related to your intensity level'. Generally, he cautioned against doing more than 15 sets per body part.

Although 8x8 was the rep scheme Vince advocated in his only published book, at various times he advocated others including 10x10 (which he, and not the Germans of 'German volume training' fame, appears to have invented), 6x6, 10-8-6-15 and 15x4. It's worth saying that for all of the rep schemes above, apart from the 10-8-6-15, the weight was supposed to remain the same throughout. Cumulative fatigue, rather than the load per se, will stimulate hypertrophy. If you can finish all the sets, increase the load next time. As far as rest between sets goes, keep it to an absolute minimum, perhaps 30 seconds or even less. In the 10-8-6-15 scheme, you perform 10 reps with 50% of the weight you will use for 6 reps, 8 reps with 75% of the 6-rep weight, 6 reps with a weight you can handle for 6 good quality reps, and then 15 reps with 35% of the 6-rep weight. The 8x8 and 6x6 appear to have evolved out of Vince's early use of the 10x10 scheme, which, as a whole-body programme, proved to be too fatiguing for many of his trainees.

Vince also favoured compound sets. Simply take two or four exercises for a given body part and perform them in succession with minimal rest between. Another intensification technique was 'burns', the idea being to maximise the pump at the end of a set by doing three or four extra partial-range reps. Not every exercise benefitted from burns, but 'ideal exercises to use burns on are Scott curls, calf raises, chins, and dips.'

Early on in his career, Vince wrote a much-misunderstood article entitled 'Muscle Confusion', the meaning of which he had to clarify more than once over the following decades. Vince was not suggesting a bastard Crossfit-style approach of never performing the same workout twice – having a different WOD every day of the year. Instead, he meant that, because your body 'does not respond to the same workout every workout session', you must pay attention to this and react accordingly: alter the tempo, reps, sets and combinations of exercises until your body does respond in the right way. Knowing what this means comes only with experience and paying close attention when exercising, something many if not most never do. For Vince, the ultimate principle was to listen to your body and to understand how it responds to training; the various schemes and techniques he came up with were simply tools to be used to stimulate the muscles in different ways at different times. None of his routines was intended to be the be-all-and-end-all of muscle building.

I've saved what I consider to be the best for last: Vince's ideas about nutrition. 'Bodybuilding is 85 percent nutrition' – this is one of his most famous maxims. In fact, he was one of the earliest bodybuilders to realise the true importance of proper nutrition and to advocate for various forms of supplementation, including among other things, liver and kelp tablets, orchic tissue (bull's testicles, also a favourite of a certain otherwise exclusively herb-eating Austrian politician), brewer's yeast, amino-acid tablets and the first commercially available protein powders.[2] Although Vince is best known for his 36-eggs-a-day diet, especially because of the recent work of raw egg nationalists like myself, the variety of his diets is actually quite great, and repays careful attention. Above all, Vince emphasised that his different diets should serve different purposes, and should only be adopted for as long as a particular purpose was being pursued. A Hollywood starlet looking to slim down for her latest role has no business slonking 36 raw eggs a day, for instance. Likewise, his Maximum Definition diet, a species of ketogenic diet, should be used for competition preparation, not for packing on mass. Even as late as the publication of *The Wild Physique*, Vince believed that 'the average bodybuilder vastly underestimates the value of diet and overestimates how good his own eating program is.'

Vince was one of the first to emphasise the need to maintain a positive nitrogen balance when building muscle.

---

[2] For details of Adolf Hitler's supplement stack, see Norman Ohler, *Blitzed: Drugs in Nazi Germany* (London, 2016).

'Protein in the body is in a constant state of exchange and must be replaced regularly if muscular gains are to be realized. This is why I recommend taking amino acids and liver tablets every three hours plus large quantities of eggs, meat, and half & half daily, to flood the tissues with a constant supply of protein.'

Constant supply of protein was one of the purposes of the 36-eggs-a-day diet but not, contrary to what the poorly-informed doctors of broscience believe, the primary one. Vince's recommendation of branch-chained amino acid tablets was part of a wider regime of pills that would make most AIDs sufferers balk; indeed, Vince was one of the first to recommend extensive supplementation, at a time when supplements were really only just beginning to become available. For instance, for the Maximum Definition diet, the following pills were to be taken: 10 amino acid and desiccated-liver tablets (every three hours); 1 vitamin C and 5 calcium tablets (every three hours); 4 orchic tissue tablets (before and after workouts); 5-10 grams of arginine and ornithine, 3-5 grams of tryptophan and 10 calcium tablets (before retiring to bed, on an empty stomach). One of the strangest diets Vince experimented with is known as the liver pill diet, which he claimed could add an inch on your arms without any extra work. In its early form, it involved taking two liver pills every hour for two weeks, but by the time of *The Wild Physique*, Vince was suggesting 50-100 liver tablets a day.

Vince did not necessarily advocate a high protein diet all the time, though. He believed, for instance, that under high stress a person should substitute high-protein foods, with an excess of phosphorus, for a lacto-vegetarian diet (fruits, nuts, vegetables and dairy products) to allow the nerves to recover and the body's calcium-phosphorus ratio to return to a proper balance. More fundamental than his sensible recommendation that different diets must serve different purposes was his belief that, ultimately, every person's metabolism is different. A person must learn their 'body's rhythms', 'because only you can determine what diets and foods are best for you'.

With only one or two exceptions, such as Chet Yorton, through the 1940s, '50s and '60s Vince was the only real bodybuilder practising and recommending what have come to be known as ketogenic diets, of which his Maximum Definition diet, used for contest preparation, was an example.

'Personally, I prefer to use fats as energy sources over carbohydrates since they sustain the body's blood-sugar level for up to six hours and as fuel sources burn slowly. In fact, due to the difficulty the body has in breaking fats down into energy, it actually burns body fat in the process.'

As I mentioned earlier, the Maximum Definition diet involves eating steak and as many eggs as you want, three times a day, with a carbohydrate rich meal, without protein, once every four days. Vince's advocacy of ketogenic dieting was not merely anecdotal but supported by serious reading, including scientific papers and also accounts of explorers like Vilhjalmur Stefansson who had spent time with the Inuit, observing and following their high fat and protein diet. Vince may also have been familiar with a paper published in the 1960s on the diet of the nineteenth-century mountain men, which detailed their high protein and high fat diet, in the manner of the Native Americans.

The Maximum Definition diet can also be an intermittent fasting diet if you schedule the meals appropriately. For instance, if you eat your final meal of the day at 7pm and then wait until 11am, you're effectively following a 16:8 fast, with a 16-hour fast and an 8-hour eating window.

Vince also recommended short total fasts, of up to five days, to cleanse the body of toxins. Chuck Sipes was another rare bodybuilder of the Golden Age who experimented with fasting, touting its restorative powers, which today would be referred to as 'autophagy'. The idea is that by forcing the body to consume its own cells by restricting food intake, newer healthier cells are produced, bringing a feeling of increased vitality. Vince anticipated another more recent trend by advocating the eating of raw foods to ensure the preservation of vital compounds including enzymes and minerals that would otherwise be destroyed by heating.

The 36-eggs-a-day-diet, or 'Hormone Precursor' diet is a mass-building, rather than a contest preparation, diet. The purpose of the diet is not just to provide a ready flow of the highest-quality protein but also a massive infusion of cholesterol, consumption of which has been proven to have a closer correlation with lean muscle growth than protein consumption has; Vince claimed, famously, that a cycle of 36 eggs a day could have the same anabolic effects as a cycle of steroids.[3] The diet involves building up to eating 36 eggs a day, in raw form, as a series of three

---

[3] See for instance the work of Dr Steve Reichman at Texas A&M University on the relationship between cholesterol consumption and muscle growth. It took two years of fighting for Dr Reichman to have his research published.

shakes. I call them 'anabolic custard': 12 raw eggs and half a litre of half-and-half (milk and cream in a 1:1 ratio); protein powder can also be added to the shake, which in the Golden Age would have meant Rheo Blair's protein powder. Vince advocated 'fertilised' eggs, which basically means free-range, not battery, eggs. Of course, as you'd expect, he was aware that the nutritional quality of eggs depends on the quality of the animals that lay them.

Vince recommended that the cycle should take eight weeks. It would look like this:

Week one: shake for breakfast; 1lb meat and salad for lunch; 1lb meat and salad for dinner.

Week two: shake for breakfast; 1lb meat and salad for lunch; another shake as a snack; 1lb meat and salad for dinner.

Weeks three to six: shake for breakfast; 1lb meat and salad for lunch; another shake as a snack; 1lb meat and salad for dinner; a third shake.

Week seven: same as week two.

Week eight: same as week one.

As with the Maximum Definition diet, Vince suggested having some supplemental carbs, in this case twice a week, on a Wednesday and a Saturday, with one of the meals. He recommended whole grain carbs such as oats, rice, pasta and potatoes. There was also a laundry list of pills to be consumed: 1 multivitamin, 1 zinc tablet, 5 alfalfa tablets, 10 kelp tablets, 3 wheatgerm tablets, 1 RNA-DNA tablet, 1 HCL tablet, 3 digestive tablets, 3 lysine tablets and 3 multi-glandular tablets. He also suggested taking 10 liver tablets every three hours, 5 yeast tablets with each protein drink, 4 orchic tissue tablets before and after each workout, and 6 tryptophan and calcium tablets before bed.

Vince used this diet himself and with his students, including Larry Scott and probably Arnold too, and again, his claims about its efficacy were not just anecdotal. He knew that at the beginning of the 20th century, it had been common practice to give burns victims a diet of 36 eggs a day, in various forms, not only raw (in shakes or ice cream or even mixed with wine) but also cooked, to counter the terrible muscle wastage that results from burn damage to soft tissue. Two studies from the mid-1960s, again which he may have read, suggested that the massive egg consumption had been mimicking the effects of newly available steroids like dianabol, which by that time had replaced the egg diet for burns victims in hospital.

Beside the hormonal benefits and the positive nitrogen balance, one of the main recommendations of this diet is the ease with which you can consume a massive amount of calories. Each shake works out at roughly 1800 calories, so in weeks three to six you'll be taking in 5400 calories from the shakes alone; with the meat meals included, you're looking at close to 7000 calories a day. As I say in my book *Raw Egg Nationalism in Theory and Practice*, pity the Virgin Meal Prepper, with his endless succession of bland pre-cooked meals!

So now you know Vince Gironda a little better than you did before, we can finally ask these vital questions: Why are people drawing pictures of Vince Gironda? And what do they mean?

Let's find out!

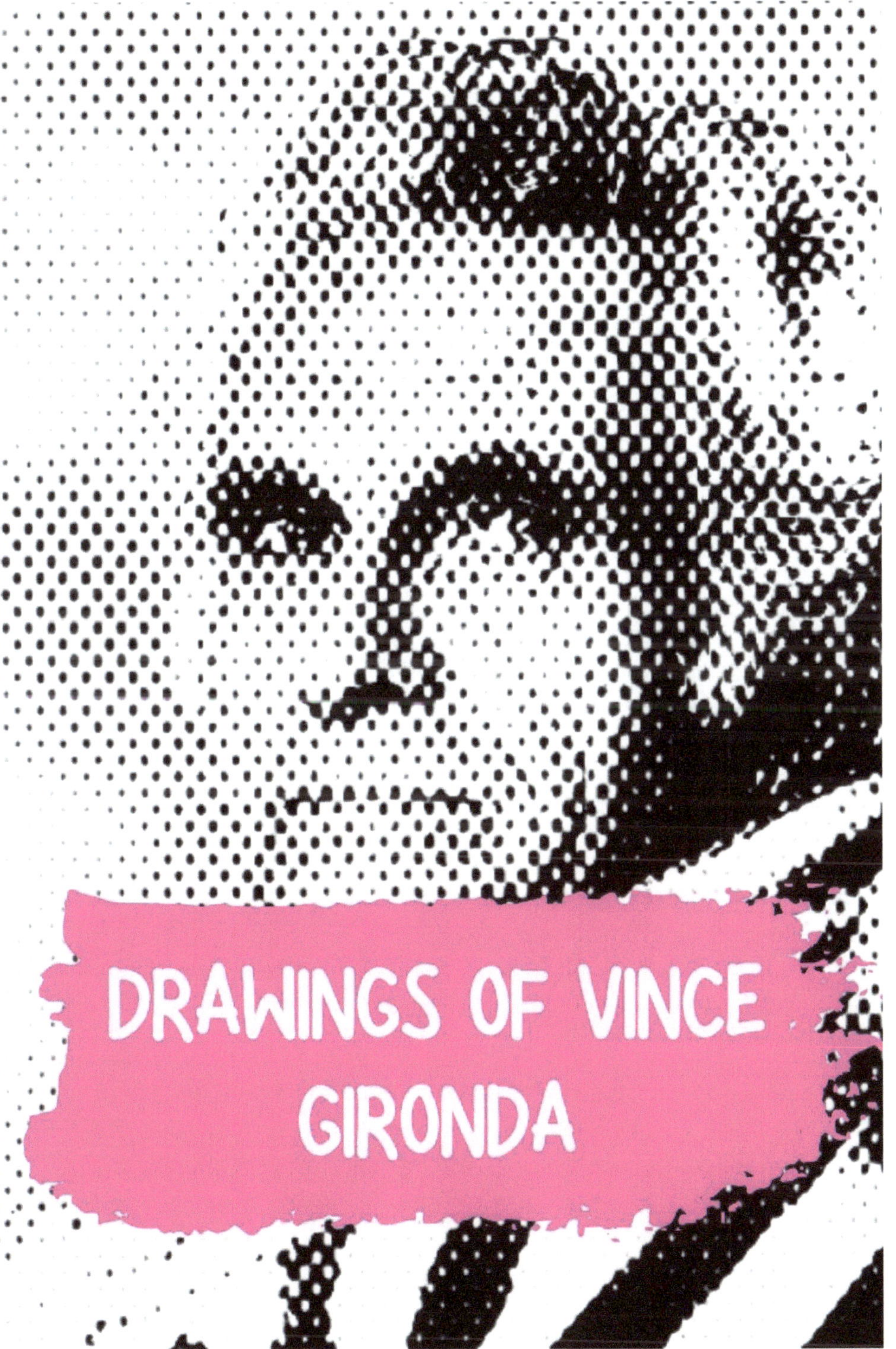
DRAWINGS OF VINCE GIRONDA

Now we all know a little more about Vince, we can get down to the very important business of understanding how to decipher drawings of him. Ultimately, interpreting Girondas is an art, not a science; you will only get better through practice and trial and error. While some things will be obvious – will literally jump off the page, as it were – others will be more subtle, and only after time will you realise their true significance. That being said, I'll try to outline a few general principles of interpreting Girondas before we get to look at some examples together.

First of all ask: is it actually a picture of Vince Gironda? Remember that I described Vince as the Nikola Tesla of bodybuilding? Sadly, he is not anywhere near as well-known as he should be, and although many young women are crazy about Vince and know all about him, others will draw you a picture of Vince Taylor or, heaven forbid, something or someone even further removed from the world of Golden Age bodybuilding. An inability to follow a basic command says a lot about a person, I think we can agree.

Second, if she actually has managed to draw a picture of Vince Gironda and not Vince McMahon, look at the period of Vince's career she has chosen. Has she chosen an image from the end of Vince's career? This may tell you that she has been contemplating deeper questions of life and death; perhaps she is of a philosophical or even morbid disposition. If she has chosen an image from Vince's glory days, by contrast, when he was at his physical peak, this suggests instead a healthy fascination with beauty and power – what we might even call a Classical or pagan mindset. Sometimes, you may even be lucky enough to receive an image from an apocryphal period of Vince's career – such as his days as a swashbuckling pirate, or his turn as a Columbo-like super sleuth investigating murders in the otherwise paradisiacal setting of 1950s Venice Beach. The artist's imagination will be her sole limitation here.

Third question: has she added any extra symbolism to the image? Deciphering this symbolism will help you to build on any conclusions you've already reached on the basis of the period of Vince's career the artist has chosen. While the meaning of everyday objects may be more or less clear, be aware that even the most mundane object can have two or more meanings. The symbolism of less familiar or exotic objects may require extensive consultation in historical, anthropological or hermetic texts. And what is Vince doing? Has she drawn a classic image of him; or has she used her imagination to place him in some unfamiliar or unusual situation? For example, if she has placed Vince in a squat rack – something Vince was known to detest – this may suggest a desire to flout convention, a rebellious streak, even a distaste for or rejection of his ideas.

Fourth, a broader consideration of the style will be necessary. Has she chosen to render the style of the Old Masters? She's obvious a classy girl, with classic tastes, not to mention talented if she manages to pull it off. Or has she drawn the image with crayons in the manner of a toddler? Don't mistake a deliberately 'naïve' style, like that of the modernists, for an inability to paint or draw. Such a deliberately naïve style will tell you a great deal about her aesthetic tastes and ultimately her character. A preference for abstraction and the reduction of the human form to simple shapes may suggest a contempt for beauty and nature. Equally, don't be too generous if the picture looks like it really has been drawn by a child. She's either much younger than she says she is – tread carefully, anon – or she just lacks any artistic talent whatsoever. In both cases, important inferences can be drawn. The use of colour is also important. A black-and-white colour palette may simply indicate that she has copied a black-and-white image, which is not in itself indicative of anything other than a preference for classic images of the Iron Guru. Other colours, for instance a prevalence of pinks, may indicate an attempt to render Vince as a gender-fluid figure, possibly on the basis of his early interest in dance. This is to be resisted firmly.

As I said, these principles are not intended to be exhaustive. Only time and habituation will reveal the subtler principles of interpreting such pictures.

So, without further ado, let's look at some Girondas I've received in recent months from young women looking to win my heart.

Not a promising start. This Gironda appears to have been abusing steroids and lifting heavy, resulting in a thick midsection of the sort that Vince denigrated in the strongest terms. The artist clearly has little understanding of the fundamental aesthetic principles Vince followed. But at least she hasn't drawn Vince Vaughan; which is to say, I don't *think* she has...

My verdict: must try harder. You're going to have to give her a serious education on Vince before you progress any further.

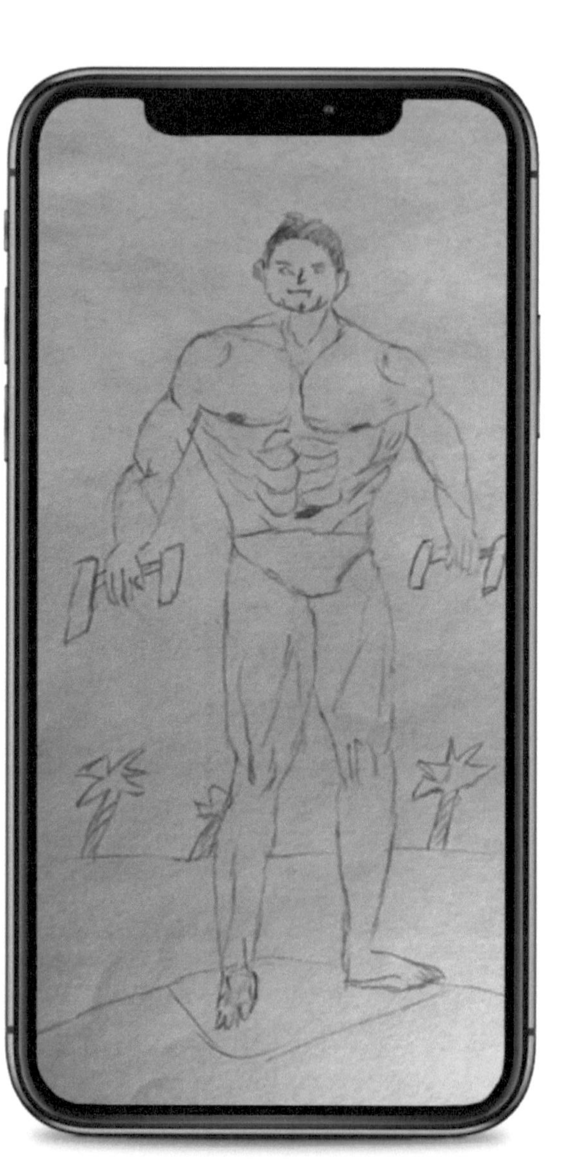

How refreshing! This is a very striking reimagining of the Iron Guru in the Andy Warhol style. A number of potential interpretations suggest themselves, but for me the most compelling one concerns Vince's rightful place in history. Warhol painted some of the most famous people of the age, including Marilyn Monroe, Elvis, Marlon Brando and Chairman Mao, so perhaps the artist is hoping to elevate Vince to the status of a great icon of the twentieth century too. I'd certainly like to think so. This suggests a nobleness of spirit and a sense of justice, as well as a creative mind and artistic flair. Good girl.

The colour scheme is also suggestive. Yellow is of course the colour of sunshine and vitality, hope and joy. The negative associations of yellow, particularly with cowardice, are obviously not to be entertained.

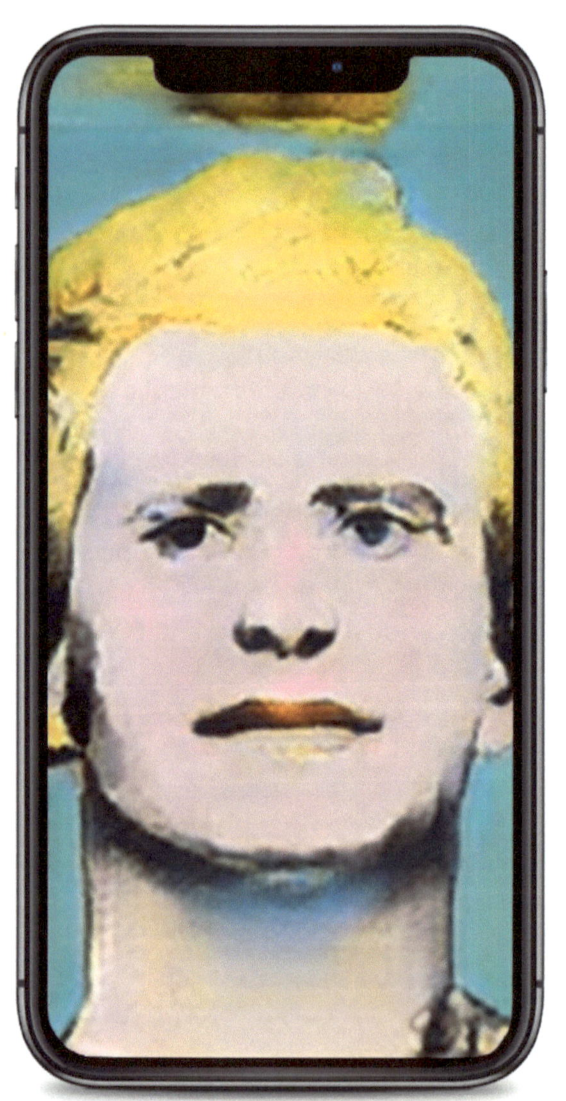

What can I say but beware the woman who says she prefers a 'dadbod'? No woman in her right mind would prefer an overweight, out-of-shape Vince (which never actually existed) to the classically perfect aesthetic he displayed in the picture upon which this travesty is based. In a rare moment of honesty, a woman like the woman who drew this may even admit why she wants you to be rounder, more approachable and less 'alpha': you make her feel fat, unhealthy and unworthy of your affection. In short, she knows she isn't good enough, and wants to punish you for it rather than changing herself. Prefer the woman who wants you to be at the height of your powers and encourages you to be so.

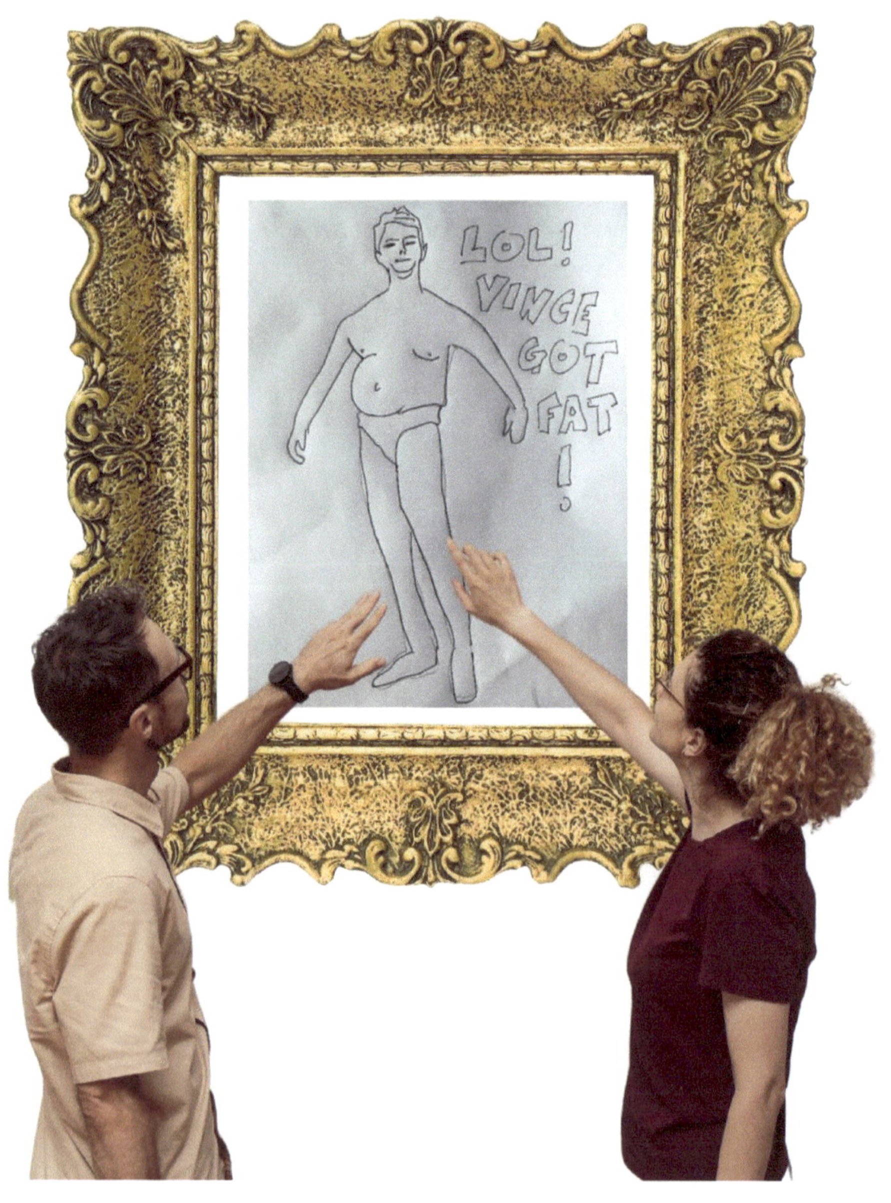
LOL!
VINCE
GOT
FAT
!

Pay attention! This young woman was obviously talking to Josh Newton Jr. at the same time as she was talking to me. Perhaps she sent him the Gironda she was supposed to have drawn for me? Well, if this drawing of a gorilla is anything to go by, it can't have been very good. Notice the lack of detail, the faltering unconnected lines and the misspelling of 'banana'. I would diagnose a general lack of confidence, as well as of learning – and fidelity.

If you want to understand the very serious art of interpreting gorilla drawings, I suggest you read Josh's fine book, *Draw Me a Gorilla*, available from Amazon.

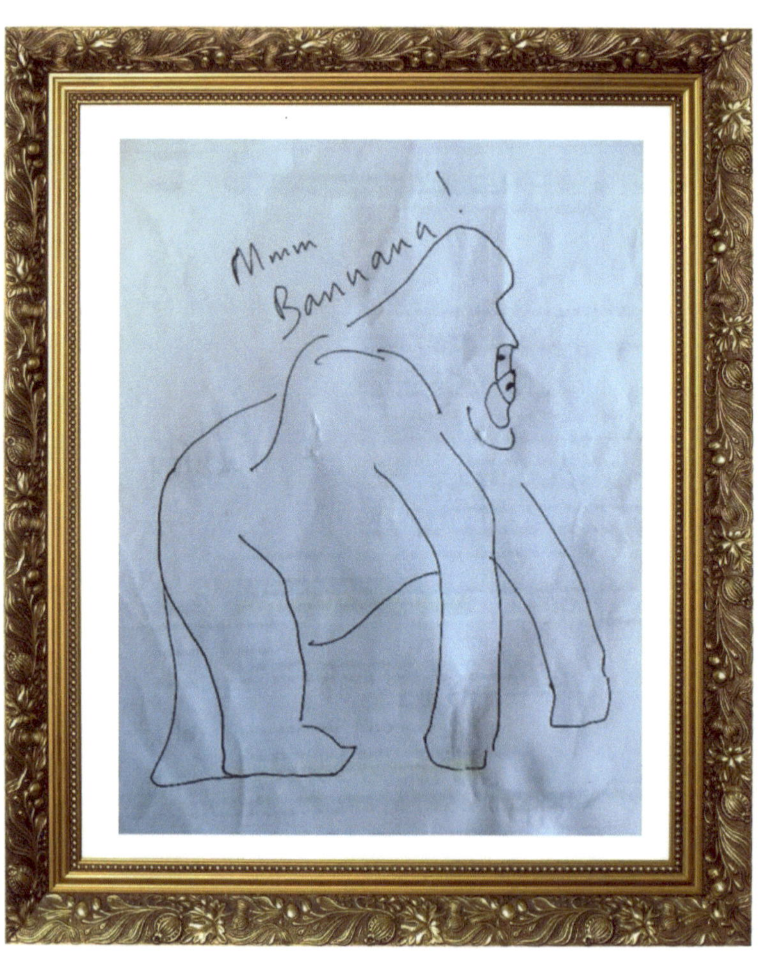
Mmm
Bannana!

There is something strange and unnerving about this Gironda – stylised, abstract, archetypal. Perhaps the artist is gesturing towards some idealised notion of the male form; but then she has chosen the wrong civilisation, and the wrong ideal. The stylisation suggests an African fetish idol – the sort of thing you'd see carved in dark wood – not an American bodybuilding idol. As much as Gironda believed the human body was a gift from God, a work of art which should be judged according to the eternal principles of aesthetics, as a good Catholic boy he certainly didn't go in for idolatry.

The eyes, in particular, are very disconcerting: empty, soulless, alien. The artist is almost certainly prey to some reptilian traits herself.

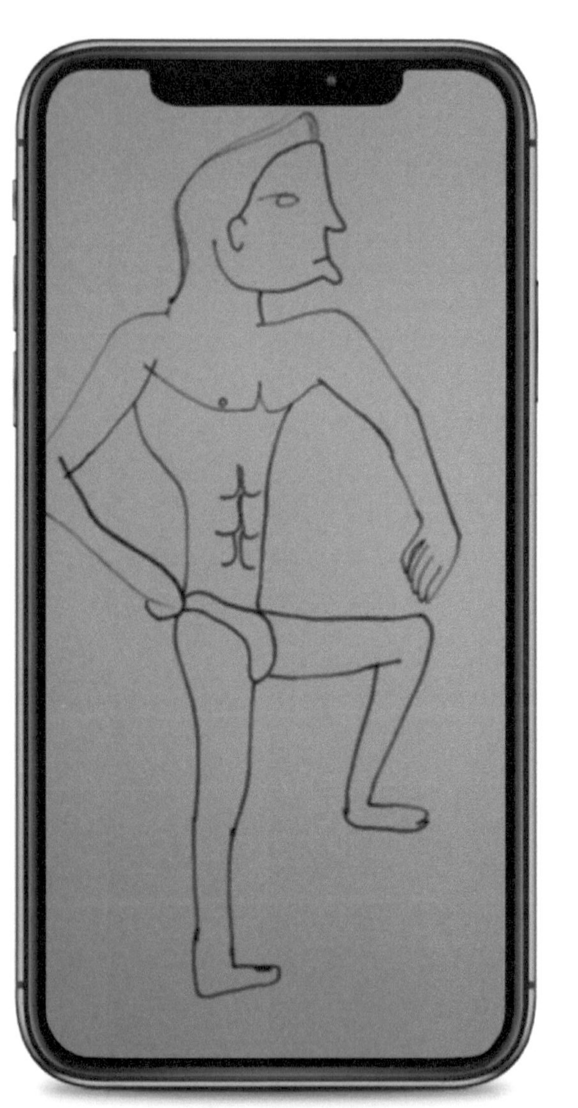

Oh dear! Another mistake! Photorealistic pencil sketch or not, this is a picture of Larry Scott and not Vince Gironda! Some mitigation is afforded by the fact that Vince trained Larry and was responsible for his transformation into the first Mr Olympia; one name is seldom mentioned without the other. Still, if she can mistake Larry Scott for Vince, what other crucial mistakes will she make? And do you want to be the one to find out?

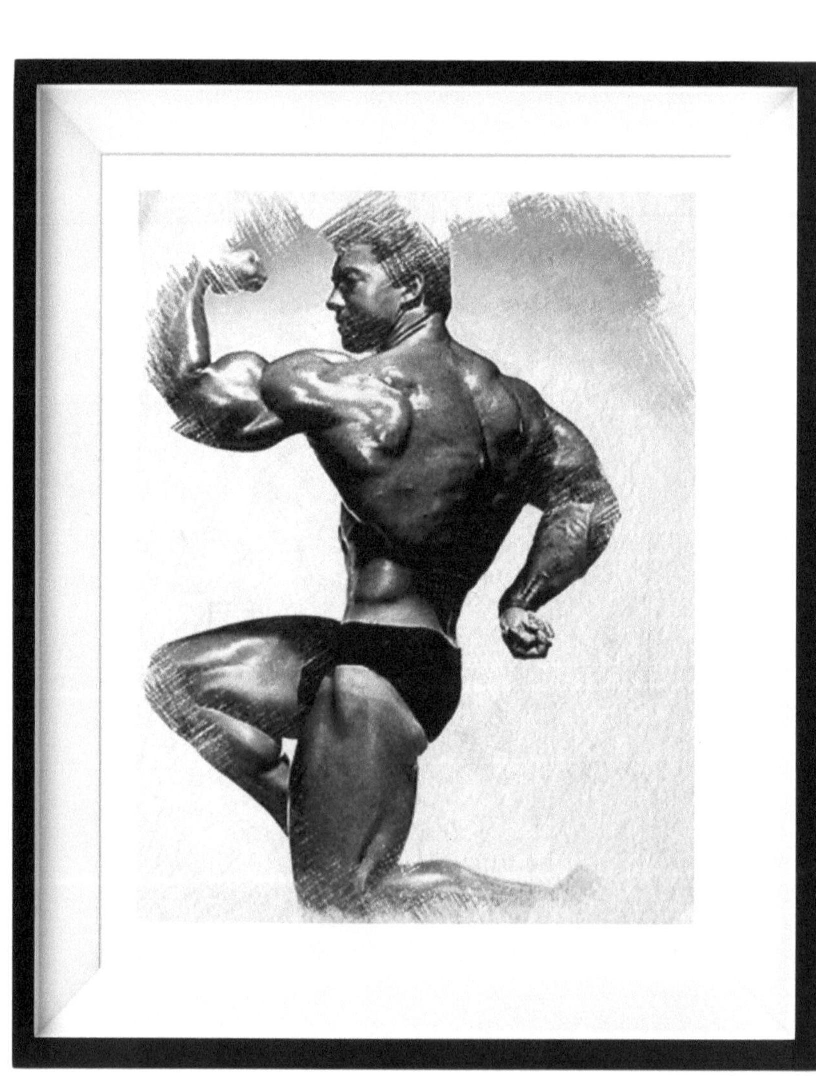

Now this is more like it! The classic Gironda. Vince as he should and will be remembered. This girl gets it. Need I say more? Go get her!

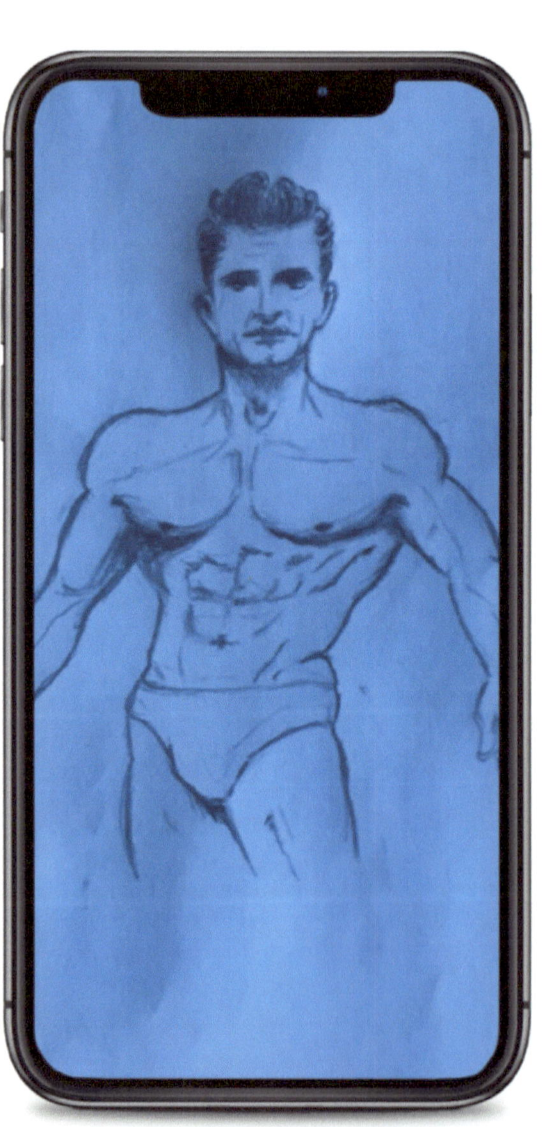

Another impressive attempt at a portrait of Vince, this time in the style, I assume, of Egon Schiele or some other figurative painter. (It's quite heartening to know that some women are willing to devote so much time to my requests to draw me a Gironda. There still is hope, it would seem.) This raw, intense image captures, I think, some of Vince's primal power, and also some of the darkness, the anger, in him too.

He has the rough air of a pugilist in this image, and an ancient pugilist at that; perhaps the artist is gesturing to the roots of the Gironda family in Italy? Clearly, the artist is an intense person herself, devoted to understanding and capturing the essence and the history of the people she studies – and that includes you too, anon.

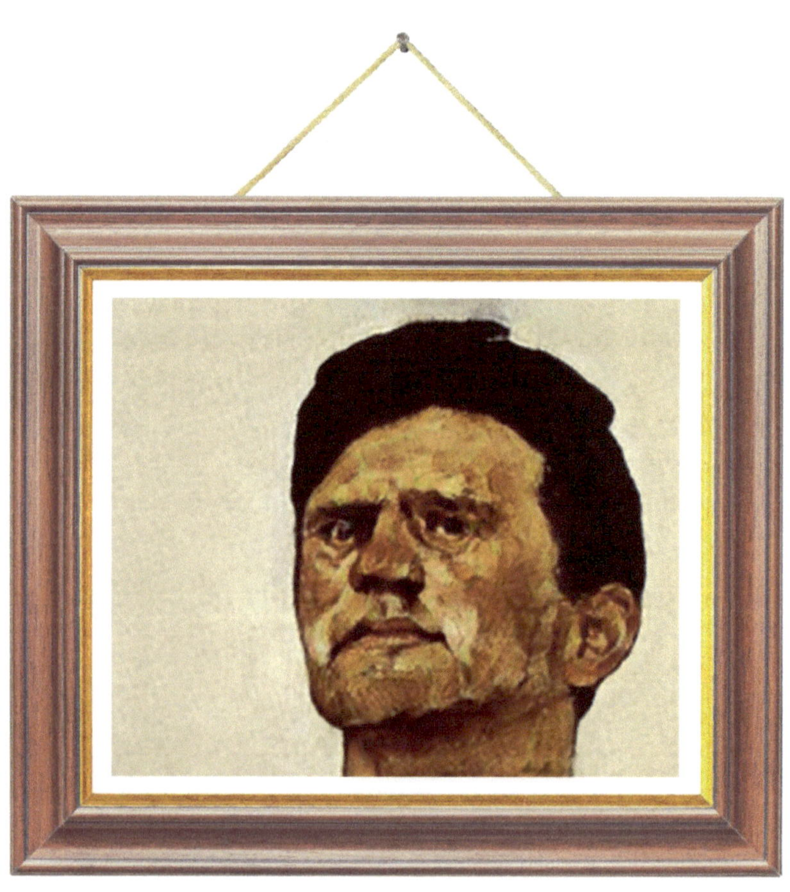

familiar-looking man enters kitchen

What are you doing?

Oh. Uh. Nothing?

How old are you, anon?

I'm uh....

So tell me then, anon, why did you ask a minor to draw you a picture of Vince Gironda?

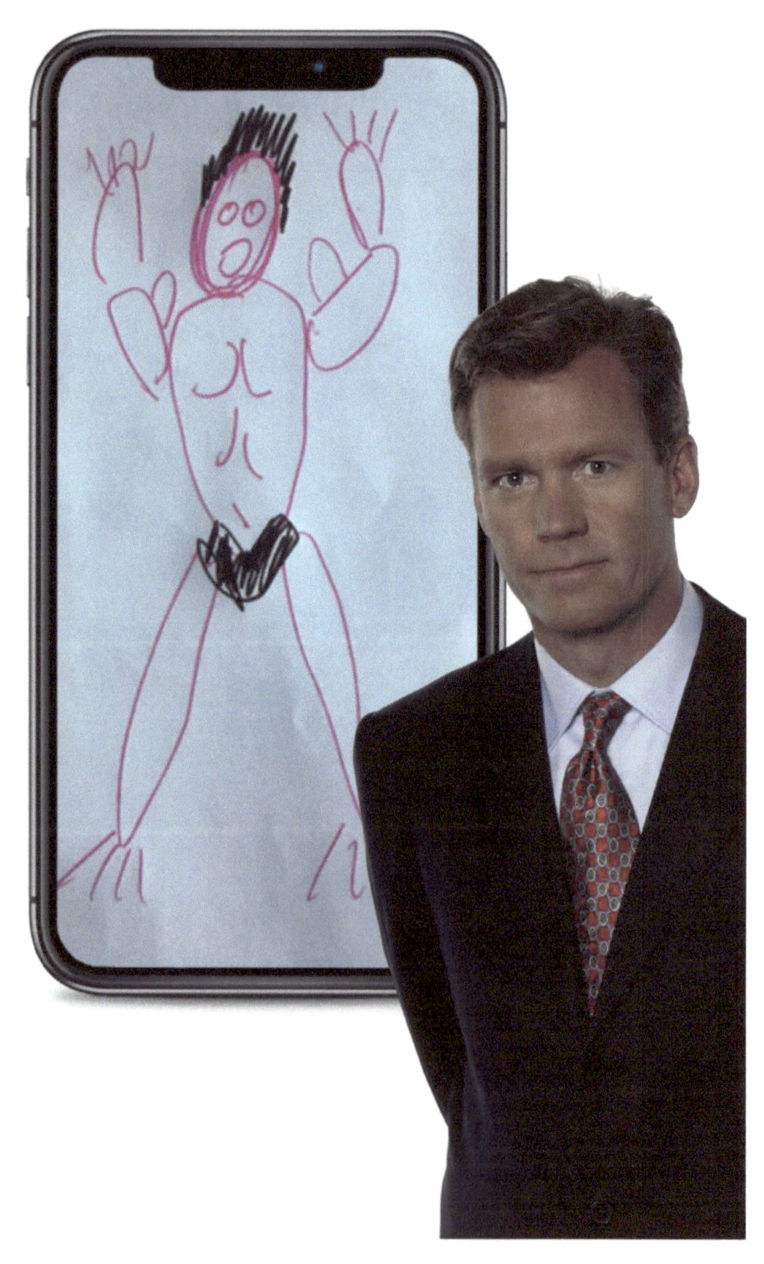

Not only has the artist chosen one of Vince's finer, classically influenced poses, but those red glowing eyes… Could it be that she's a raw egg nationalist herself? Well, what are you waiting for, anon? Ask her!

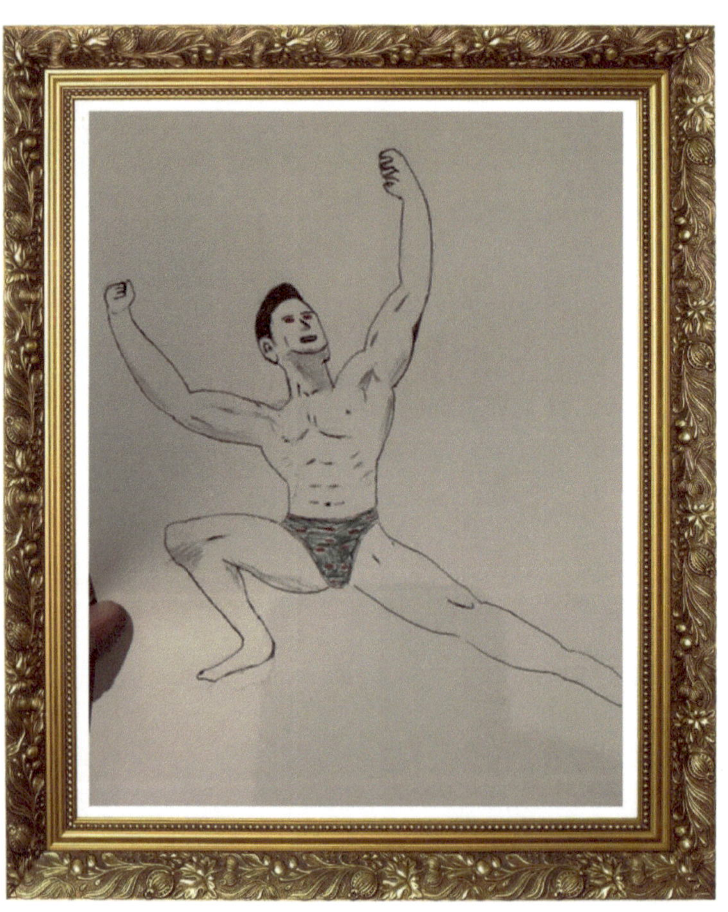

Here we have the same pose as in the last drawing but, boy, what a difference! Gone is the beautifully proportioned body and the elegant pose; this Gironda could be an irate English builder on the beach in Spain, cursing a seagull that has just stolen his bacon sandwich. Diagnosis: anger issues, feelings of impotence.

Another source of worry is the fact that the artist has given Vince a cloven hoof instead of a right foot, a clear suggestion of satanic influence.

The replacement of the mouth with a sausage may have obvious Freudian significance.

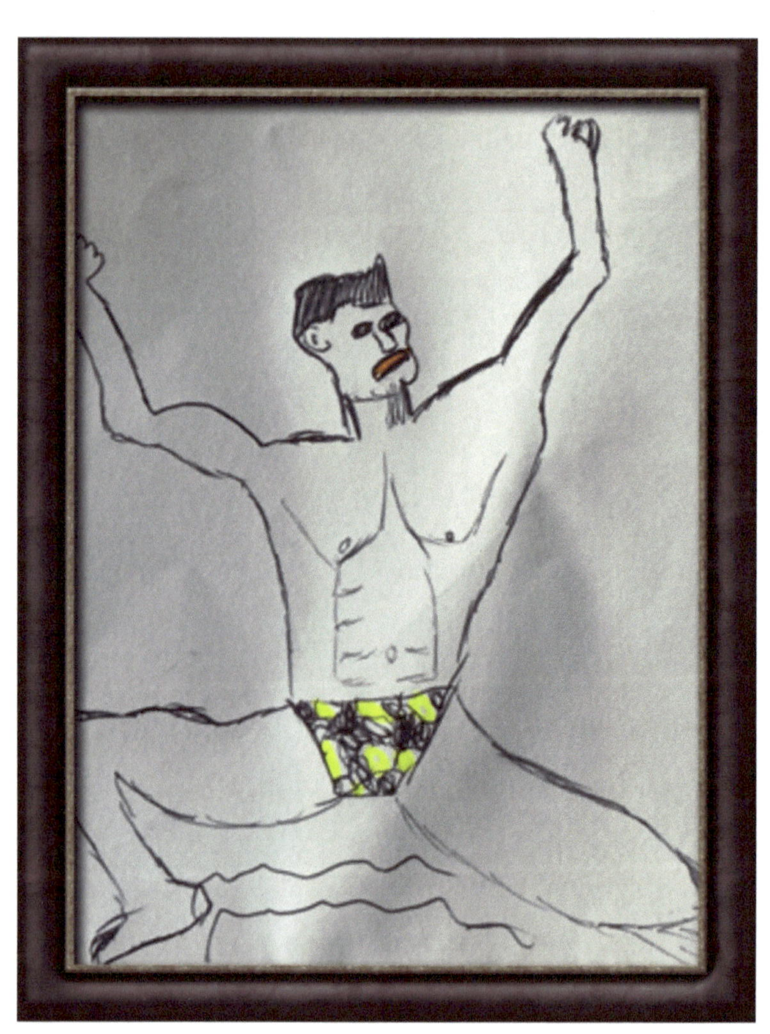

This Gironda has more the look of an Abercrombie model – the sort who stands in a doorway all day posing for photographs with giddy young Asian girls – than the Iron Guru.

The proportions are wrong: this Gironda clearly hasn't been following Vince's advice about the careful placement of mass. For one thing, unlike Larry Scott, this chap has naturally broad shoulders, so he shouldn't be afraid to develop his traps more than he has. Nothing, unfortunately – short of becoming a mass monster, one of Vince's pet hates – will balance the sheer size of his head, and not even the Maximum Definition diet could shrink it. Confused.

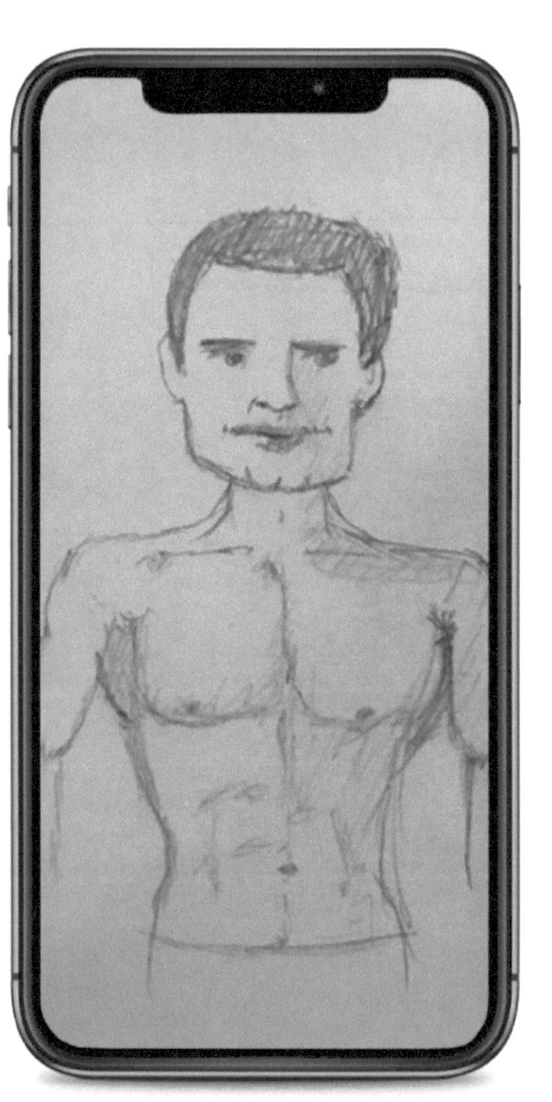

I spoke too soon. *This* is confused. Holy moly. I can only assume, and this is me at my most charitable, that this nightmare vision is some attempt at a riff on one of Vince's patented exercises, the sissy squat. I've already said that this is actually a very taxing exercise, even if only light weights are used; it's definitely not for sissies. (Why the exercise actually acquired that name is a mystery to me. Perhaps it's because it looks a little bit like an overenthusiastic curtsy, something Vince would never, ever have done.)

All good charity aside, this Gironda can only be a window onto a deranged mind. The question is, how long are you going to look through it before you turn tail and run?

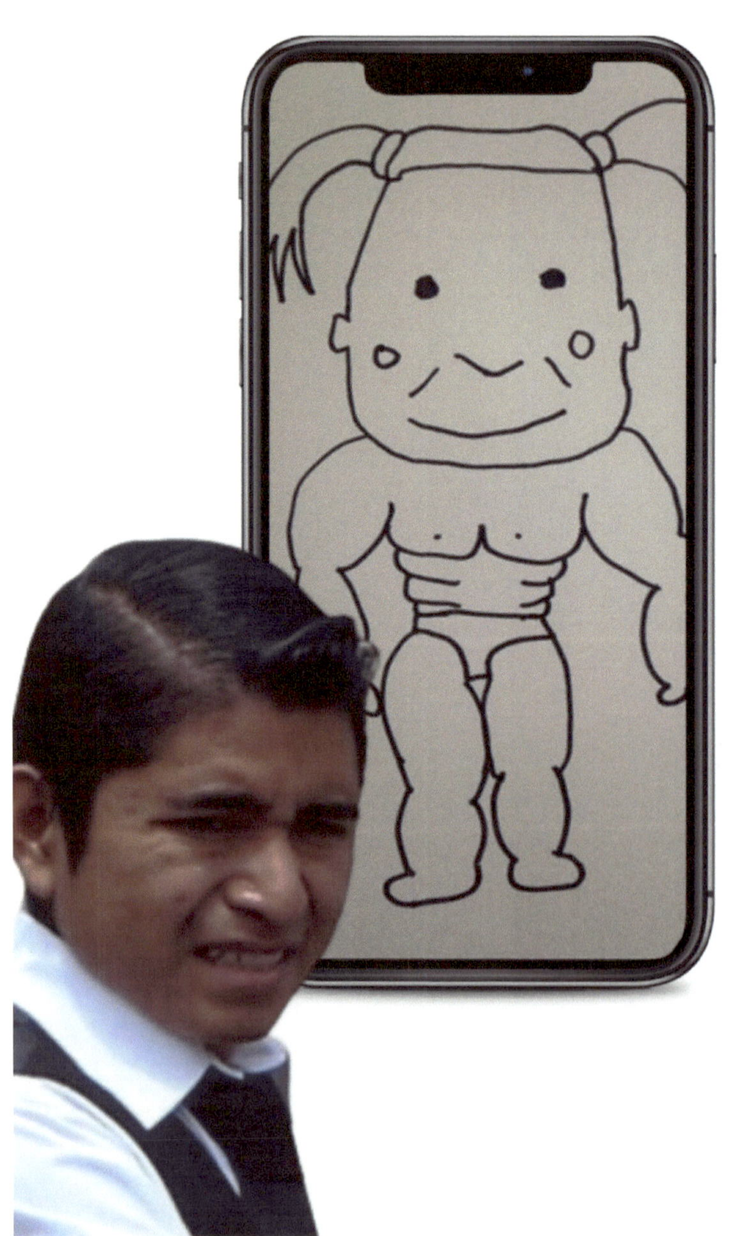

DRAW YOUR OWN GIRONDA

Now is your opportunity to practise drawing your own Gironda. Take your time, don't rush. Try to draw something authentic, whatever comes to mind, rather than drawing something you think will prove some point or other about you. It's easy to tell an inauthentic Gironda from an honest one: there's a reason Vince's most famous workout is known as the Honest Workout.

Once you've finished drawing your Gironda, take a look and analyse it. What do you think the drawing says about you? Does it tell you something about yourself you didn't know before?

Drawing Girondas can be great therapy. If you're feeling stressed, draw a Gironda. If you're feeling low, draw a Gironda. If you're feeling elated… Whatever your emotion, let it flow through the pencil or pen or crayon or whatever tool you're using. Externalise your feelings in Vince. Assemble an entire sketchbook full of Girondas drawn at different times, in different moods. Looking back, you'll be surprised at just how accurate a record of your life these drawings provide. If you want, Tweet your favourite @ me (@babygravy9).

www.ingramcontent.com/pod-product-compliance
Lightning Source LLC
Chambersburg PA
CBHW040259240726
48664CB00006B/1309